# CANCER TREATMENT
## A practical guide

What you need to know and
nobody tells you.

### Gillian Howell

ISBN:
9781699349120

## DEDICATION

To D, D, R, and K

# CONTENTS

# ACKNOWLEDGMENTS

All that I know has been taught to me by the amazing, dedicated healers and brave people I have met along the way.
Thank you all.

D, you are irreplaceable x

# The Cancer Journey an introduction

This is a journey nobody wants to go on, but according to statistics one in three of us will set out on this journey at some time. Some even say that up to fifty percent of the population may do so as we live longer and avoid other illnesses. This inevitably means that everyone in our western society will experience cancer very personally, either directly as a patient, or through a close loved one.

As time has gone on treatments have continuously improved with success rates being achieved that were only dreamt of twenty or even ten years ago. The treatments themselves are much softer and more precisely targeted with less side effects than ever before, but cancer remains a taboo subject, shrouded in fear and secrecy.

Because of our reluctance to discuss this topic, virtually everyone embarking on this journey finds that they feel isolated and frightened.

This book is kept brief and easy to read, and will tell you the things you need to know. You will find out what is normal, what to expect and when to seek help. By telling you what happens and how to prepare for each stage of the journey, you will have realistic expectations and therefore be able to plan and manage your treatment and recovery.

# 1
# Bad News
## The Initial Shock.

Some people develop a growing suspicion that "There is something not quite right", for others it comes like a comet out of the blue.

However it comes, it is almost inevitable that you will find yourself in a room with an "expert" delivering a diagnosis and projections. The professionals deal with this situation daily and they talk their own language. Their world is full of words that are strange to the lay person, which, combined with our own experience and worries, adds to the fear attached to already frightening words such as; surgery, chemotherapy and radiotherapy. Any one of these is liable to send us into a panicked tail spin where words merge into each other.

Typically, the professional continues to talk studiously avoiding eye contact, then ushers you out of the office into a completely changed world. You may have been left hanging or passed to another professional, but all you know, as you rush down the corridor, eyes averted, is that your world has changed and you need the sanctuary of home.

This interview and diagnosis represents all our fears in one hit and can be so overwhelming that our brain simply stops functioning and we plummet into the state of extreme shock.

Shock is a primeval reaction, hard wired into our brains rather like a rabbit caught in the glare of oncoming headlights. Shock manifests itself in many ways and you may experience some or all of them.

They can include;

- Weakness of limbs, legs may be wobbly and unsupportive, arms weak.

- Eyesight may become blurred with difficulty focusing.

- Nausea or even vomiting.

- Feeling disorientated, dissociated, "in a bubble".

- Understanding may decrease with words not making sense or "holding".

- Dizziness or fainting

- Gasping or sobbing

All of these in a mild form are normal and to be expected. However, a big shock can lead to serious complications which will require help. Here are some conditions you need to be aware of

### Respiratory Complications.

Your breathing may initially, as mentioned above become laboured, perhaps gasping as if someone threw cold water in your face. If this continues, becomes distressing or if you have an underlying chest condition you would be wise to seek medical help.

### Heart Complications

We now have greater understanding of heart distress and the signs and symptoms of a "heart attack" have become more understood. They can include;

- Chest pain - pressure, tightness, squeezing;

- Pain - as well as pain travelling from the chest to the arms (either ,but usually the left), jaw, neck back and abdomen may also be affected;

- Dizzy or light headed;

- Sweating;

- Shortness of breath;

- Nausea, vomiting;

- An overwhelming sense of anxiety or "not right(ness)";

- Coughing or wheezing.

As you can see the symptoms are not clear cut and the expression "Heart Attack" can be misleading. For many, especially women, the elderly and diabetics, myocardial infarction, where the heart tissue is damaged, is a process rather than an event. Sometimes with little pain but a strong feeling of something very wrong. In retrospect a pattern can often be uncovered but if it feels wrong get medical advice. You have had a severe shock and are under a lot of stress.

**Stroke**

It would be foolish to discuss heart complications without mentioning the signs and symptoms of a stroke which everyone should know as general knowledge. In the United Kingdom the national health service runs a campaign called "FAST".

**F**    Facial drooping - unable to smile or stick the tongue out straight

**A**    Arm weakness

**S**    Speech difficulty

**T**    Time, is crucial, call emergency services get help.

Once you get home and begin to feel safe the adrenaline that got you home dissipates and shock deepens.

You will need a quiet, darkened room to rest and recover. Try and remember to sip water frequently to keep hydrated. Sugary snacks can help too

Your mind has received a terrible blow and activated its automatic response by going into the state of deep shock. It needs to close down and conserve energy to rebuild itself. Just as your computer freezes and needs to reboot, your brain will close out external stimuli and unnecessary energy expenditure to do the same thing.

In humans of course, vital processes need to continue to sustain life, but non vital areas will be affected. Everyone is different and has different tolerance levels and you may experience some, none, or most of the symptoms of shock to various degrees. This stage usually lasts around twelve to twenty four hours.

You should also be alert to the fact that, as explained previously, shock can uncover another underlying illness or disorder which may also need to be addressed. There is a difference between not wanting to do something or mild discomfort which is normal and inability, pain and distress which will need medical advice.

During this period of your brain trying to reorganise and reboot you might experience;

• Mental or emotional numbness,

• A reluctance to tolerate bright light or difficulty focusing,

• A reluctance to tolerate noise,

• Wanting to be alone and not bothered,

- A mild headache is normal but unusually severe pain may be symptomatic of a deeper problem and will need medical advice,

- Weakness and exhaustion,

- Digestive disturbances - reflux, acidity, lack of appetite, nausea or sugar cravings,

- Sleep disturbances - unable to sleep, vivid dreams.

Please note that any cardiac or respiratory symptoms should have rapidly resolved as these are vital for life and not symptoms of shock.

Metaphorically speaking, your mind has received a serious blow and is retreating to the "back of the cave" where it feels safe to rest and recover. You need peace and quiet to think, process and accept this new reality.

As you feel stronger and begin to recover, your mind will tentatively venture 'back out' and into the hustle and bustle of daily life. Time is the best healer and it will take as long as it takes, but here are some tools you might like to try:

- Homeopathy -
  Arnica is especially good for shock. Arnica 30 can be obtained over the counter from a pharmacist. Suck one tablet four times a day,

- Rescue remedy -
  Bach flower remedy. Easily obtained over the counter,

- Mindfulness and mind calming apps,

- Calming music.

We all react differently. And during this period issues can arise over physical contact. Some like to be held by their loved ones and to comfort each other during this stage, but others can find it overwhelming and too much stimulation. It can be difficult if the affected person does not want physical comfort and the loved ones want to express their support in this way. Of course you are all deeply affected by this illness but just now the the needs of the patient must come first.

Please try to see this as just a reaction and not a rejection. Closeness will return later. There is a section devoted to partners and family further along in this book.

As the initial shock recedes your brain will begin to recover and the enormity of the situation will begins to sink in. The brain is still low on energy, so the first thoughts will probably be negative ones simply because these take next to no energy to contemplate. We always think the worst when we are stressed and tired. More positive feelings will return as recovery progresses.

The whole process can be illustrated in a simple diagram:

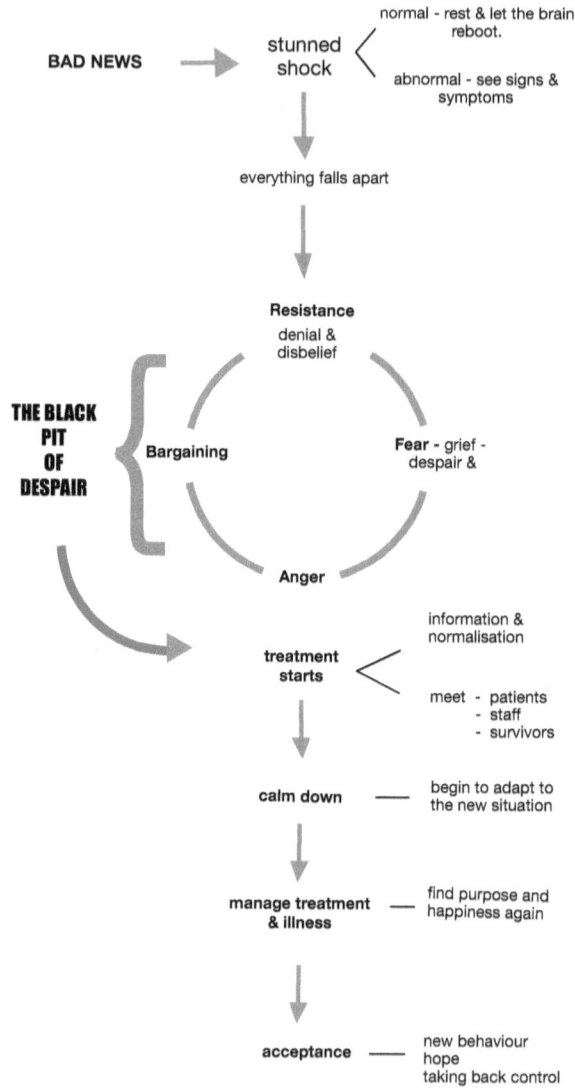

After diagnosis one feels as if one is falling apart. This leads into the period of "stunned shock" which can easily aggravate another underlying condition so it is necessary to know what is normal and what is not.

Soon the brain, like any machine will begin the "start up" process. There is very little energy available at first and thoughts which use the least energy come first - these, of course are the negative ones. Our ability to process is still compromised and it is easy to fall into the cycle of distress.

## The Cycle of Distress

Falling into the cycle of distress is horribly easy, not just after the initial shock of diagnosis, but at anytime, especially when you are overtired or simply overwhelmed by it all. I think all of us have experienced this state at some point in our lives when we have been severely challenged, and the cancer journey is one of the biggest challenges of all.
After diagnosis and stunned shock comes;

## Denial, disbelief

First we resist by denial and disbelief. We simply cannot accept that this has happened. Why me? What have I ever done? The results are wrong. They got the names mixed up. It'll all be fine, just ignore it. I feel fine. These are the very normal low energy rationalisations as the brain struggles with the enormity of this new situation and does not want to accept the challenge. It wants to turn the clock back to a happier place.

## Grief, Depression.

As realisation dawns there is a great sense of loss. All the things that, at this time, you may feel you have lost. The carefree days stretching endlessly into the distance. The happy times. This is a particularly negative and incorrect state which can fall into a black pit of despair. There will be happy times ahead, but at this stage you simply do not have the energy to see beyond the diagnosis.

## Fear

Fear hits hard and heavy and is behind a lot of this negative thinking. Cancer is scary and hospitals are scary. The perceived loss of control is especially scary.

## Anger

Anger can be a good starting point in many situations to help pull you out of distress. It requires energy and is higher up the emotional scale. If recognised and used correctly it can act as a springboard to spur you into action. However, all too often we become whipped up in it. "The doctors are idiots", "It's all this (or that) persons fault."

It is strangely appealing to waste hard gleaned energy and fall into a state of impotent fury which often ends up developing into jealousy of the unaffected and deep SELF PITY, which although understandable and totally warranted, is a deceptively dangerous place that saps all positivity and healing ability.

## Bargaining

"I'll give this up or do this thing and all will be well." Energy is used up railing about the unfairness and bargaining for a better outcome. Soon all the energy is used up and one may fall back into denial, hopelessness, loss of faith, self pity and down into the black pit of despair.

All of these horrible negative emotions are normal and are symptoms of a bruised and exhausted mind. Ultimately it is your strength returning and treatment starting that enables you to regain the control which will pull you out of this terrible cycle.

Depression, as well as being a symptom of over tiredness, is further discussed later in the book under "Churchill's Black Dog".

The LESS ATTENTION you give negative feelings, the SOONER they will pass. As time goes on you will learn more about your condition which will help you to understand and combat negative moods. Just now, as you do not have the information, try to keep busy and distracted.

This waiting period is very difficult. Not knowing what lies ahead is terrifying and the imagination can run riot. Once you get the full picture and things begin to happen you will regain control of your life again.

Fortunately, this is a short time although it seems long going through it. I would love to give you an easy solution for this period but, so far, none has been forthcoming. The best I can suggest is to be kind to yourself and try not to let your mind run away. Few things are ever as bad as first thought. It will pass.

Once a treatment plan is formulated the medical team step in and things will begin to happen very quickly.

This is very good on two levels;
On the purely physical plane the sooner treatment starts the better for obvious reasons. On the mental plane it finally gives you clarity and allows you to regain control as you become more knowledgeable and meet others undergoing the same journey.

You will begin to calm down as you realise things are now being done and you are not alone. Soon, you will realise that you have accepted this new state and are actually working with the medical team. By having realistic expectations and an understanding of each stage of the process you will find you are able to manage your progress, and before long, begin to find reasons to smile and enjoy life again.

# 2
# GETING READY FOR TREATMENT

This journey is the most challenging thing most of us will ever do in our lives. How we choose to approach it will make an amazing difference to both the experience and to the outcome.

As the initial shock recedes the medical team step in with startling efficiency filled with procedures and plans.

It is normal to be frightened. Hospitals are terrifying places filled with sharp implements and monstrous machines. You will find yourself in a strange and alien place which seems to have no similarity to your previous existence. It smells different and looks different. Time has little meaning here and everyone seems so busy and purposeful it's hard to know where you fit in and what you are supposed to do.

Everyone feels like this at first. It takes a lot of courage to show up for that first appointment, and if you can do that, you can do the rest!.

Knowledge is the best weapon to fight fear. By choosing to become engaged with your treatment you will learn what the medical team are trying to achieve and how they plan to do it. This will give you a realistic understanding of your treatment plan so that you will be prepared and will understand each step of your journey and any "bumps" that might occur along the way.

I am sorry to admit that the professionals are not always as good at sharing information as we would like them to be or indeed as they should be. It is easy for them to forget that each patient is going through this for the first time and needs to hear the fundamentals. Please ask. No matter how silly it may appear to you, it isn't and it is good for the professionals to get grounded again.

Another good tip is to take a note book, ask and record what side effects you might expect, what to do and when and where to go to get further advice. Some areas such as the UK NHS use the family GP as first contact in most situations, whereas other regimes have direct contact or partnership arrangements. Make sure you have all relevant contact details, inside and out of hours before you start treatment.

Hospital staff are generally happy to talk and fellow sufferers can be very supportive, especially those who area a little further along the treatment route to yourself. By talking to others you will develop realistic expectations. Many of those will meet will have experienced side effects or set backs and may be able to share coping tips. Very few people will complete the typical pathway of surgery, chemotherapy and radiotherapy without at least one poor blood result or a surprise infection causing a set back. Talking to others and sharing your story will help everyone.

**Include your loved ones**

Cancer diagnosis does not just affect you but also your loved ones. Many people feel guilty for bringing all this pain to their families and try to protect their loved ones by avoiding the issue and pretending nothing has changed. This is a slippery slope which can isolate the whole family as everyone tip-toes around the "elephant in the room".

Not everyone feels comfortable having personal conversations and this can be quite a challenge. If you feel this, perhaps talking to a trusted member of the family and asking them pass on the information until everyone becomes more accepting of this new reality will help.

We humans are a very adaptable species and even though we resist change we can actually cope with it very well. Once everyone is aware of what is going on and that they are allowed to talk about it, they can "come on board" and support both you and each other along this difficult path.

**Mental health**

It is widely accepted that depression is a symptom of cancer. Not just because cancer is a lot to deal with but it is also thought to be an actual physiological symptom.

So, you have a double whammy to deal with; cancer and depression. This makes fostering that all important positive attitude a daily challenge.

To actively consider how we feel and take measures to improve our positivity is a new concept to most people. Western society tends to be reactive and to dwell on negativity. For example, how many of us start the day with a news program telling us of the latest disasters and political intrigue? News shows are after all, just shows competing for ratings like any other.

The sad fact is, negative stuff attracts more people than positive. Which is interesting when you think of it isn't it? Many have written as to the hows and whys if you want to investigate further, but just for now, let's simply accept this as a fact and think about becoming more positive.

First and foremost, avoid unnecessary stressful situations. There are things which must be faced but worrying about the state of the nation will not help! As you progress, be selective of those you spend time with. If they are moaners and grumblers or make you feel down - move on. Life is too short. One of the most amazing and unexpected things about this journey is the wonderful people you will meet who make fabulous companions and role models.

**Mindfulness**

Mindfulness is a modern buzz word. People talk of it as if it is something new, but it's not, it is just a modern technique of meditation, a practice as old as the hills. From ancient times we have realised the power of controlling our minds by learning to cut out needless distractions and focus our thoughts.

There are many ways to learn; books, apps, local groups and teachers. Mindfulness and meditation are extremely beneficial as they create a clear healing space. Letting go of the worries and clutter of daily life and becoming centred allows you to find peace within. As well as feeling great this allows your brain to redirect energy away from pointless stress towards healing.

$$F_{(Focus)} + I_{(Intent)} = O_{(OUTCOME)}$$

Focus plus intent equals outcome. In other words, if you want it and think about it, you will find ways to make it happen. Some call this formula the secret of life. Mindfulness is one tool, active positive thinking is another.

Thinking positively is an art and a skill which improves with practice. We are creatures of habit, often falling into negative thought patterns without even realising. Poor thought patterns, like any other bad habit can be changed, but it takes effort.

### Be your own best friend

Remember to be kind to yourself and treat yourself as your very best friend, which you are. Actively seek things you like. A walk in the park, coffee with loved ones, lovely music.

There will be black times; what Winston Churchill described as his "Black Dog Days" will happen. Plan for these in the up times by developing an "exit strategy "such as, for example, "When this happens I will give it 10 minutes of focused negativity (use a timer!), then I will get up and make a cup of tea or walk around the garden."

It is normal and necessary to visit our fears. By doing this we can achieve understanding and formulate plans. However, dwelling on things helps no one.


**Create a Sanctuary**

Before starting treatment look around your environment and plan a little sanctuary. You may wish to remove things that are liable to make you feel sad or stressed. Think of, perhaps, a nice comfortable chair with a foot rest, an easy to reach table with a light where you can rest surrounded with photographs and memories that make you smile as you recover from surgery and further treatments.

You might like to be near a window and put up a net curtain so that you can sit in privacy.

Try compiling a lovely music list that you can listen to when feeling sleepless or having a down day.

A thermos flask is always a useful addition so the drink of your choice is always available.

Some people like to set up the spare room. When returning from surgery partners often cannot sleep for fear of bumping or jostling their loved ones during the night. Also, after an anaesthetic, aside from the surgery, most people find their sleep patterns very disturbed with naps rather than a deep sleep so it is nice to have your own bed where you can rest or put on lights or music without disturbing your partner.

Think of comfort foods to put in your freezer or stock up on you favourite chocolate biscuits, this is not the time to calorie count!

Perhaps you would like to re organise your 'phone. Think of who you want on speed dial, perhaps change the call ringtones of friends and family so that you know those you need to answer and those you need not.

There will be a lot of pills! Think about how you are going to store them both safely and accessibly. Some people choose to include a lockable chest on a nearby table easily reached but also safe from little fingers.

By planning in advance you will have things the way you like them without leaving it to others to guess or creating an unwanted fuss.

# 3
# TREATMENT

Treatment regimes are, of necessity, tailored to each case. This chapter is therefore very general with some tips that may help as you prepare for this stage.

**Going into hospital for several days**

Personal pride and a little style go a long way to keeping your spirits up so treat yourself to a lovely new dressing gown or robe to wrap up in. New, easy to walk in slippers and gowns or pyjamas made of cotton will keep you feeling fresh. Bring a lap blanket for sitting out and add your own pillow, in a coloured slip to avoid confusion, for comfort.

Bt taking the time to make the effort to look as good as possible every day you will enhance your self esteem and your recovery rate. So ladies, remember your make up and gents your grooming kits. Skin gets very dry in hospital so add moisturisers, lip balms and hand cream. Dry shampoo spray is also helpful as hair washing is not always possible every day. Remember, however, that storage is always a problem in hospital, so pack small containers.

**The day centre**

Day Centres do everything from minor operations to delivering chemotherapy.

As procedures and anaesthetics improve, many operations, which took days or even weeks in hospital in the past, now allow you to go home in the evening where you will more comfortable and less stressed therefore shortening your recovery time. You will be told what you are allowed to eat or drink prior to admission and need only pack a small bag with night wear and basic toiletries. Space is usually an issue, so wear light cloths which are easily put on keeping in mind where your wound will be.

**Getting home**

You will need help, so bring a loved one with you to keep you company while waiting. They are usually advised to go home whilst you are in surgery and in the recovery room as you will be asleep. The hospital will either ring or advise them when to return. Ask them to pop a couple of pillows and a blanket into the car for your return journey.

You may feel very excited when you get home but this is just a release of tension and bed really is the best place for you. Let your loved one do all the ringing and telling, tomorrow is another day!

Our society does not understand the need for rest and there is an a lot of pressure to just go back to normal. However, all procedures are a great shock to the body, even the seemingly small ones. Especially in this field where there is so much worry and anxiety.

Immediately after any surgery you will be running on adrenalin and chemicals. These will dissipate over the coming days and, as they do there will often be an upset and often weepy period. These are natural stages as the body and mind adjusts.

Recovery can be difficult and sleep patterns are often disturbed. Plan your pain killers for maximum effect when you want to sleep. Read the instructions and take the painkillers as recommended even though it may seem a lot. Pain is much easier to control if it is kept at bay and suffering pain is not helpful as it stresses the body and slows healing. There are some further helpful hints in the "Side Effects" chapter. As you improve and the soft tissue heals you will find you are able comfortably decrease the dosages.

The first 3-4 days following surgery are the most painful as the soft tissue recovers and swelling subsides. Most people note a distinct improvement on days 4-5 .

**Chemotherapy**

The initial appointment which involves locating a blood vessel and deciding the mode of delivery is usually the most active. Many people have a long term portal installed which allows easy reconnections. These are often around the collarbone and held in place by a small stitch with the connection end shut off between treatments. They need to be kept scrupulously clean and dry to prevent infection, so reading the care instructions and following them to the letter is crucial.

After that receiving chemo is rather like a long haul flight with long tedious periods of sitting waiting for the IV's to deliver. It is an exercise in being 'a patient patient'. Ease discomfort by choosing loose comfortable clothes with loose sleeves and necklines. Try bringing a "care bag" along with such things as a cushion, slippers, lap blanket, earphones, eye mask, snacks, favoured drink and entertainment such as a tablet or book. It is also during this time that you will meet amazing, inspiring people, some who will become friends for life.

**Radiotherapy**

The radiotherapy experience is totally different to the serene chemo department. It is busy, bustling and very scientific. On your first appointment you will be "marked out" and "blocked" to expose the treatment area and protect surrounding tissue. This may also include a bespoke shield which will take time to make. The first time you see the machines can be quite daunting and there may be a lot of positioning to get the angle just right. After that it is just in and out, often every day for a number of weeks. There is no sensation during exposure and the sessions are short. Timing is of course crucial as this determines the dose received.

It is easy to begin to feel a little frustrated and dehumanised during this process but this is not the intent. It is simply a product of the short treatment times, the level of accuracy and the frequency of delivery necessary. Although frustrating, it really is worth it to spend what may seem like a long time waiting for such a short exposure.

Radiotherapy often comes as the last treatment on the cancer journey and can appear to be a long tiresome period to be tolerated. However, human beings are amazing and you will soon find yourself settling into the routine. The waiting room can be quite a sociable place. Wear comfortable clothes that can be quickly removed and replaced and bring an appropriate care bag with perhaps a gel cushion!

# 4.

# SIDE EFFECTS
# AND HELPFUL TIPS

Cancer treatments are an essentially destructive process designed to target the cancer, destroy all irregular cells and prevent their spread. They are very strong and unfortunately they produce side effects. The hospital staff will discuss these with you so that you know what to expect at each stage.  There are some that are almost inevitable.


**Hair loss**

This is the most dreaded side effect as people feel it marks them as a cancer patient. This is a shocking experience for both men and women and there is no easy way through this.  Cutting or shaving hair early can make you feel more in control and avoid the upset of clumps of hair falling out.

Another, often surprising symptom of hair loss is how cold you feel without your head being insulated. Head wear such as hats or scarves are popular.

Many patients wear a silk or cotton cap underneath to avoid irritation and for warmth. Wigs are popular but again can be uncomfortable to wear for long periods.

Dressing with care will also help your self esteem. So try manicuring your nails, both men and women, even if you never did before. It's amazing how such a small thing can help you feel groomed and attractive. The extroverts among us revel in big jewellery, strong make up and crazy hats and wigs. Try not to become disheartened and remind yourself it is only for a short time. Your hair will begin to grow again as soon as chemo stops - sometimes with surprising results.

**Nausea and sickness**

This is common, especially after the chemotherapy sessions. This can make you feel miserable. The team will discuss this with you and do everything they can to minimise the symptoms. You will need help to get home safely where you can lie down. Many organisations offer free transport for both chemotherapy and radiotherapy sessions run by an army of volunteers who tend to be very lovely and supportive people.

Aromatherapy treatment, such as 2 or 3 drops of mint oil to 6 drops of lemon, inhaled either on a tissue tucked under your pillow or placed in an aromatherapy diffuser can help.

The staff should have discussed with you the dangers and symptoms of dehydration and should provide guidelines. If not, ask them what they consider normal, and make a note and recored who and when to call and for medical help. Keep these in mind and call for help sooner rather than later. Often all that is needed is a simple injection and a sleep to be able to start drinking, and feeling better, again.

**Weakness.**

This is progressive throughout treatment and will be discussed in the "What happens after treatment" section of this book. Just for now be aware of it creeping up. You will not have the energy to do the things you did last month. This is normal and a sign of the destructive effects of the treatment progressing. Try not to over do things or become frustrated with yourself. It is necessary for your recovery and it will pass.

**Skin care.**

Unusual allergies and skin sensitivity are common affects. Choose natural fabrics if possible and avoid scented cosmetics as much as possible.

A major irritant is biological detergent. Non biological detergents are easily obtained and a double rinse cycle can also help if you find your skin very sensitive. Fabric softeners are also best avoided as they add a chemical coating to the fibres to make them feel soft but this also interferes with absorption.

During radiotherapy certain skin products such as soaps and creams can actually burn under the treatment. The hospital staff will give you a list of safe products to use.

## Infections.

As you progress through treatment your immune system will weaken leaving you prone to infections. This is a necessary part of the process to kill the cancer cells, but unfortunately it affects the whole body. Keep this is mind and avoid exposure to coughs, colds and heavily populated places. Even taking all the care you can, infections can still sometimes happen causing delays in your treatment program. Try to catch them as early as possible when they are most easily treated. A thermometer is a good tool - and act quickly.

Discomforts such as over heating or becoming chilled, over tiredness and emotional distress will also take their toll on your immune system because they use up valuable energy.

## Mouth Ulcers

If you are unlucky enough to suffer from mouth ulcers, which are another common side effect, it will take effort to remember to drink, but it will pay off.

This is a miserable stage. It will pass and the tips below may help you through it:

Notify your medical team if mouth problems increase. The sooner they can detect a complication the easier it is to treat.

- Keep your mouth clean. Use a soft, or child's, toothbrush and brush morning, night and after eating. If you wear dentures clean them thoroughly. Remember to disinfect your toothbrush by placing it in boiling water. Just put it in a mug filled with boiling water and leave it until the next time.

  Flossing, or anything which will encourage your gums to bleed is to be avoided. This is because the amount of blood platelets, which are necessary for blood clotting, is lowered during treatment. This means small lesions can be hard to heal and may lead to a very red, sore mouth that is open to infection. Your medical team will prescribe an analgesic mouth wash or foam if your mouth is sore. In extreme cases an analgesic IV can be deployed.

- Dryness. Try to keep your mouth moist as dryness will encourage fungal growth. You may also be given anti-fungal lozenges or drops to help combat this problem. It is very important that you use them regularly as fungal infections establish themselves and increase rapidly. Avoid acidic drinks and even regular toothpaste can sting.

  The simple use a straw can really help.

- Oil Pulling - This is an ancient practice which is completely harmless and can leave your mouth feeling very comfortable. It works on the idea that oil dissolves and "pulls" out all bacteria in and around the mouth. This is done by swishing oil, coconut or sunflower for example, but any mild oil seems to work, around your mouth for as long as you can and then spitting it out. Do not swallow because it is now believed to be full of harmful toxins. Experienced oil pullers can swish for 5 - 10 minutes. I can manage about 1 minute, but I do think my mouth feels better. Look it up on the internet for more details if it appeals to you.

## Diet

Your body is concentrating on the battle at hand and pouring all its resources into the battle field. Reinforcements (food) are very necessary but digestion takes energy which will temporarily detract from the front line fight. Therefore, it is wiser to nibble nutritious food throughout the day than to overload your body with a heavy meal. If you eat too heavily, and that may not be very much as time progresses, energy needed for healing will be redirected to your gut causing nausea, vomiting and faintness. At the very least you will feel bloated and uncomfortable.

Shakes are great and there are lots of easy recipes available to get you started. This is the time to go high calorie, so add cream, coconut milk, ice cream or whatever you like best. Try including some roughage, chia seeds and the like, which will help you combat constipation which is another side effect of lack of exercise and the medication. Remember to make them the way you like them. If they are too thick or acidic you just won't be motivated to sip them throughout the day.

Many societies traditionally advocate broth, Jewish Chicken soup and Chinese bone broth for example. Any soup made with stock from marrow bones either home made or bought will be beneficial. When you consider the destructive nature of cancer treatments on one's bone marrow to kill stray cells it makes perfect sense to replace the 'building blocks'.

Have four to six light, tasty, easily digested meals, shakes or snacks each day. Try to eat about every two hours. If you don't want to finish the meal or snack, remove it and wait until next time. Do not pressure yourself. Think fresh, tasty, comforting, and nutritious. As you improve your appetite will pick up.

Fluids are most important. You need to keep hydrated to flush out toxins from the illness and the medication. Most people just keep fresh water at hand and sip frequently.

**Sleep**

As mentioned before., expecting to sleep all night is unrealistic and sleeplessness is often a side effect of medication. The healing pattern is one that tends towards frequent napping.

The best thing you can do for yourself is simply to expect this and not get stressed out.

Sleep will return as you regain your strength and are able to stay awake for longer periods. Your body is doing what it should, pushing the limits to regain strength. You will probably be offered sleep medication and some people choose go down this route, but is really only a short term measure and can bring it's own problems later on down the line, so consider your options carefully. Many choose a middle way of occasional sleep medication to avoid dependency.

The nights can be long and lonely and it is planning that will see you through. Many people choose to continue in the same pattern as in the daytime which breaks up the long dark hours with designated snack times and use meditation and music to pass the time

## Pain control

The best tip for taking prescribed medication is to take it regularly as recommended and on time. It is very tempting to wait until pain creeps up, but it is then harder to subdue and often takes extra medication to get it back under control.
Pain is unpleasant and of no assistance at this point. It stresses the body, distracts from the healing process and makes you feel miserable.

A good tip is to set a timer to remind you when medication is due - and take it on time! As the acute stage passes you can then start to slowly and gently cut back.

As well as medication there are some other methods that can help, especially for mild breakthrough pain between medication times. However, please be sensible and don't over exert yourself. If you feel the breakthrough building please consult your medical team, pain control is something we are very good at.

*Heat.* Imagine nerves as thick electric cables made from bundles of thin fibres where some fibres within the cable can conduct electricity faster than others. Fortunately for us; within our nervous system the sensation of warmth travels faster than the sensation of pain and it can block out the sensation of pain replacing it with a comforting warmth. Heat pads on the affected area and warm baths can be very soothing. Warm, not hot, is all that is needed for this effect to work, so don't overdo it, you do not need burns!

*T.E.N.S.* (transcutaneous electrical nerve stimulation) The TENS machine is battery operated and portable. It sends mild electrical impulses through electrodes affixed to the body by sticky pads and works by confusing the pain signal in a similar way as warmth. Discuss this option with your Doctor, it is not suitable for all but it can be of assistance.

*Distraction.* Becoming interested in something else will blot out mild pain signals. Plan an interesting, low energy, activity to start about an hour before your next medication is due. Craft work such as needle work and model building can be both engrossing and satisfying.

*Meditation and relaxation.* Becoming tense always increases pain. Try a relaxation/meditation/music tape before pain is felt, perhaps during the last hour before medication is due.

## When you feel fidgety.

This is really annoying, but it is a backhanded compliment. It means you are getting well enough to feel bored – so, celebrate it! Distraction is always the cure. Keep a little store of things to do or think about when it strikes. This is a good time to write your personal journal, do a puzzle, colour in or complete some small chore. As you get stronger you will be able to do more and the frustration will pass.

## Churchill's Black Dog

Depression as mentioned before in "mental health" is an actual symptom of cancer as well as an understandable feeling. The black dog will visit, at expected and unexpected times. Most people take antidepressants during this period because the body's normal chemical reactions are compromised due to our livers and brains coping with the illness and its treatment.

There is a lot of bad press about anti-depressants, but this is only when they are over used. There is a time and a place for all things, so please consider your options carefully. A short course now can really help. As your strength returns the medical team will help you to 'wean off' if necessary. The 'weaning off' process gently reduces the medication allowing the body to return to normal production and natural balance.

**Personal journal**
This is for your eyes only. Buy a nice book or if technical, start a new folder.

It is important to be able to express our deepest darkest feelings and ever since people have been able to write they have used this outlet. Victorian ladies suppressed and frustrated, or soldiers frightened and trying to be brave have used this method as a safety valve to sanity for years.

In the dark times you can write out your frustrations and fears honestly and without judgement. This somehow helps to get them out and dilutes their strength allowing you to carry on for another day.

In the good times write all the things you are happy and grateful for; which Weill cement the positive memories, enhance the experience and prolong the feel good factor.

Some people like to read back, some page mark the good feelings, others never revisit. The choice is yours.

## Music

I really believe in the healing power of music and mention it frequently throughout this book. If you are interested in this you might like to look at the work of Dr Masaru and his work on water memory or music and it's effect on plants growing.

Music is often our way of expressing emotions so choose pieces that you resonate with and soothe your heart. It is great to have a personal play list for relaxing times and "Black Dog" days when you need up lifting.

## Crystals

These are controversial and considered a bit hippy these days. However, I, and many others use them and see positive benefits. I think of them as nature's little power packs, batteries if you like. They, like many of the alternatives, use vibrational energy to influence us. They are safe to use, lovely to look at and at the very least, what harm can they do? Plus, it is not necessary to believe to get the benefits.

Crystals are most effective closest to the skin and kept warm by your body heat. Many ladies choose items of jewellery or tuck them into their bra. (Size does not necessarily matter!) Gentlemen carry them in wallets and pockets.

Try tucking them under your pillow at night to aid sleep or leave them in the natural light of a window to influence the atmosphere of a room. When choosing a crystal look carefully and one, (or several) will "call" to you.

Sometimes crystals begin to loose their colour, this is because you have sucked out the healing energy. To re charge simply leave them in direct sunshine.

Here are some of my favourites:

Rose quartz. This is the crystal of unconditional love. Choose a smooth stone to hold and keep warm with the warmth of your body or a lump to put in a room. It draws away negative energies and replaces them with harmony and reassurance. It is a stone of deep healing. A great jewellery choice.

Amethyst. Amethyst balances out negative vibrations and is well known for its healing properties. Many like to carry a nice pointed "tooth" alongside the rose quartz.

Quartz points Clear quartz is a healing amplifier and stone of protection. As well as on your person "point out" your home or room by placing pointed "wands" at the corners of your home. "Pointing" your bed is a well known aid for restful beneficial sleep especially if troubled by nightmares.

There are many more crystals and lots of information about them both books and on line.

## Aromatherapy

Aromatherapy is a great aid for relaxation and to help support your immune system. An aromatherapy massage or oil diffuser can comfort and aid recovery. There are a lot of lovely combinations and recipes easily available from aromatherapy shops and on line. For example, I always burn a lemon and peppermint combination in my office, lemon uplifts the mood and peppermint is good for it's antimicrobial properties. Together they keep the air clean, discourage nausea, enhance positivity and support the immune system.

For night time, there are pillow sprays and many relaxing combinations for diffusers to aid relaxation and sleep.

## Flower essences

These are readily available over the counter or on line. The original Bach Flower Essences are the best known but there are other producers as well and literature available for use. Flower essences tend to concentrate on emotional states and do what they say on the label. They can be very comforting especially when the "Black Dog" visits and good to use when medication is wearing off. They are non invasive and will not interfere with your medication.

## Homeopathy

There has been a lot of great work done recently in the homeopathic word to help those suffering from cancer, support conventional medical treatment and aid recovery.

Homeopathy is a non invasive form of energetic medicine. As with all energetic disciplines, it works by aiding the body's natural defences. It takes the form of remedies usually delivered orally by a small pill or liquid. The remedy holds a particular frequency and seeks the vibration or frequencies it can aid. If it is not present, nothing happens, but if it finds a resonance, it will support it and there will be a rapid beneficial effect. Homeopathy is totally safe to take alongside your medication.

Homeopathic kits can be bought commercially. They carry clear instructions and are used by millions throughout the world on a day to day basis. They are however, as generic as the conventional medication you can buy in the pharmacies and, like conventional medicine, need prescribed prescriptions from qualified practitioners for deeper conditions.


## Acupuncture

An ancient oriental energetic healing discipline. Again, there are a lot of recent studies on it's help with cancer. Usually delivered by the use of very thin needles inserted in critical spots on the body to improve and support depleted areas.

However, for the delicate or faint hearted, acupuncture does not always involve needles and can be very effective in controlling pain and boosting the immune system.

## Alternatives
There are many more therapies and disciplines out there which could aid your recovery. Talking therapies such as hypnosis, NLP, (neuro linguistic programming) and Tapping can all be effective. Body therapies such as Chiropractic, Bowen and Osteopathy or spiritual based disciplines such as reiki are also worth considering, to give a few examples.

Talk to others and do your own research. The rule of thumb is, however, to choose a qualified practitioner and continue as long as it feels right. Most people choose a variety of disciplines and dip back and forth as they feel is right. The healing journey can be a long one and it is up to you whom you choose to see and when. We are all different and respond in different ways.

# 5

# WHAT HAPPENS AFTER TREATMENT?

Most people understand what the surgery entails because it's physical and obvious, there is a scar and then there is tenderness. It is easy to see that you need rest. Chemotherapy is also understood and people expect to be washed out and tired afterwards. The exhaustion of radiotherapy, however, generally comes as great surprise.

If you have been lucky enough to go through the whole "typical" cancer treatment of surgery, chemotherapy and radiotherapy without delays (which would you make you extremely unusual as most people need a break due to irregular blood results or infections), you still have a long road ahead. Your body has been severely tested and needs to recover.

The process is very similar to the recovery from mental shock. As with mental shock the brain pours all its available resources into rebuilding and prioritises those most necessary for survival. It can be roughly divided into three sections as time passes.

The nurses of old, who really understood convalescence, concentrated on rest, a stress free environment, a fresh wholesome diet and gentle exercise.

Recovering from cancer treatment takes longer than you might think, up to two years, and can be divided into several periods as the process progresses.

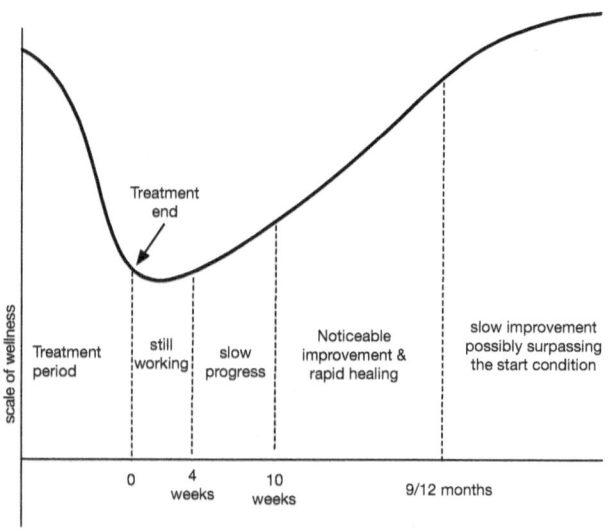

## Deep Healing Mode
(until around three months from your last treatment.)

It is wonderful to finally receive your last treatment and you have every right to be very proud of yourself. However, this is just the end of another chapter of your recovery story.

We know cancer treatments are a destructive process designed to target the cancer, destroy all irregular cells, and prevent spread. The treatment is a cumulative process and your treatment will have ended at this point because it has now reached the optimum point of effectiveness. This means it is still active and it will continue to operate. You have simply, if you like, stopped climbing up each tread of the staircase to reach the top.

You stop at the peak of effectiveness. Your body will now begin the long process of recovery as the destructive effects of the cancer treatments dwindle and your body starts to heal and renew.

This can be a very trying time and often comes unexpectedly as most people have been so looking forward to the day their treatment ends so that they can start getting their lives back to some sort of normality. The reality is that no matter how relieved you might feel to finally stop the effort and anxiety of constant hospital visits, you will also cease to receive the attention and support of the staff and fellow sufferers.

Also the positive adrenalin boost you produced to face each intervention is not needed now and will be redirected into vital healing.

This lack of contact and purpose can make people feel cast adrift. Many report feeling isolated and neglected. "I feel like I just dropped off a cliff" is a common reaction.

All the interaction stops abruptly. No trips to the hospital, no more counting down to day zero and no more delight as you cross another step off. Day zero has come and nothing (literally) happens. No great energy boost, no more having to get up and get out for appointments, just long seemingly empty days stretch ahead. Many people feel tired, fed up and disappointed. This is a very normal feeling and due to unrealistic expectations and lack of that adrenalin boost. You are very tired and your body is still fighting a hard battle.

Think, perhaps, of yourself as a weary soldier. Bruised and battered - but still here! The battlefield is a mess and the land must be rebuilt, so you have quite a job ahead of you and it will take time. First you must rest, then you need to gather your strength to start again. The land must be tilled, seeds planted and seasons to allowed pass until productivity and prosperity is restored.

This early stage is the time of repair and physical and mental exhaustion. Hours will just pass. Aid this stage by allowing rest. You know what exhausts you, so avoid it. Expect to spend long periods sleeping and on the sofa just resting.

Remember the first stage of mental shock? This is a similar rapid healing period only from a physical cause.

Loved ones are also glad treatment is over and may be desperate to do things with you to "perk you up", as to them, you might appear to have lost your will to fight. It is very well meaning but they don't understand what is happening.

Just now you need rest until strength builds and the brain decides it has healed enough of the body's vital functions to permit the expenditure of energy to external inputs. If you try to push it, your body will stop you and you will only put yourself back. This can be a frustrating and an even worrying period for all. But try to be a patient patient!   As before, it is a normal and vital part of recovery and it will pass.

Again, remember the healing powers of music. Eat lightly and often, keep warm and rest.   Many people have reported to get great comfort from watching a potted plant grow and flower or simply looking out of a window.


### Gradual Awakening
(About three to six months after finishing treatment)

After the deep healing mode you will start to "see a vague flicker of light at the end of the tunnel".

The effects of the chemotherapy and radiotherapy are mostly faded by now, so the destructive period of fighting cancer is ending.

Your energy levels are slowly building as vital processes recover but you will still be feeling a lot of weakness as your muscles begin to recover and will continue to need rest to continue healing.

Normal everyday life begins to encroach and you will start to feel interested in things again. This is because the body is now recovered sufficiently to allow energy to the mind. Many people report that they start to enjoy non energetic, but interesting activities such as reading and watching television. Interests that they may have found too much bother or irritating during the late treatment and deep healing stages.

You will start to enjoy stress-free visits, just one person at a time, and quiet chats. But remember that too much input will overwhelm your brain, which is still very occupied with the recovery process. You will experience this by fuzziness of thinking and understanding with great waves of bone deep exhaustion.

Short outings can be very beneficial, but take it slowly as many people report they find the outdoors to be vast and frightening with even thirty miles an hour feeling like a racetrack!

It's a waiting game and pace is the order of the day. It is lovely to begin to start living again and easy to get carried away in the moment and forget the danger of over tiredness which can hit hard and fast, ruining the rest of your week. Take it slowly. Accept that it takes time and learn to listen to the signals your body sends you when it is time to rest.

Please keep in mind that after chemotherapy and radiotherapy, your body's immune system needs to completely rebuild, so you are still very susceptible to infections and viruses. Even a mild illness will knock you back a long way. Avoid people with coughs and colds and highly populated places. This will come later. Just for now enjoy rediscovering what a beautiful world we live in

This is a great time to go for massages and other alternative treatments if you are not already using them as they will make you feel better and help boost the recovery of your immune system.

The nurses and healers of old, who really understood convalescence, concentrated on rest, a stress free environment, a fresh wholesome diet and gentle exercise. I don't think human beings and how we heal has changed, just our understanding. Please listen to this wise advice. It has been tried and tested over centuries. Take your time. Perhaps think of healing as building a wall. Build each layer correctly with no gaps using strong bricks and you will build a wall that will last.

### **Getting it together**
(About six months to twelve months after finishing treatment)

Around six months have passed from your last treatment you will find that you are beginning to get back to the person you were.

Although you are still not up to full strength by any means, you can see the healing process working, but it can also be very frustrating. Many people talk of "a hollowness". Looking fine on the outside but not feeling solid all through. That's because you are not fully healed yet.

**The rapid upward swing of improvement seems to tail off. So what is happening?**

Well, as far as your body is concerned you are functioning so your brain allows the thinking and processing functions more and more energy as we interact and live again. However, there is only so much energy. "Peter" must be robbed to pay "Paul", and, because in modern society we live so much in our heads, we think this is OK, which it is, but remember, there is a price.

Two things are important here;
         One, our old friend pace.
         Two, the second shock wave.

**Pace**
It is so hard to hold back when life beckons. There will be periods of frustration as you feel you are just not picking up fast enough. One just gets so sick and tired of being sick and tired!

It's a difficult balancing act and no one wants to appear vulnerable as the periods of exhaustion will still hit. Take it easy. Of course you want to do all the things you did before and "dance until midnight" but not just yet.

It's hard to refuse invitations as you look well on the outside and our society has a notoriously short memory. You will need to be patient with them as they have not been tested as you have. All they want is everything back to the way it was before and to forget the "unpleasantness".

Your immune system is recovering but you will be still be susceptible to infection and minor illnesses. As time progresses and your general health recovers your immunity will strengthen but you still need to be aware and take care of yourself.

## The second shock wave

This only happens when you are physically fit enough for it and is therefore a sort of backhanded compliment. It is nowhere as near as dramatic as the first when you received the "bad news" it but can be very deep and ultimately life changing.

A serious illness is a lot to get your head round. You have been severely tested. You have experienced loss and fear and pain. As you were recovering there simply wasn't the energy for deep thought. All your resources were focused on survival. Now, as you become physically stronger, you begin the think about what happened, the treatments you received and the relationships you experienced; those who helped, those who let you down and new people in your life.

Many people feel a deep sense of loss for that which has past, which is a type of grief and even survivors guilt for people lost along the way.

Flash backs, panic attacks, depression, nightmares and sleep disturbances may occur. This is the mind trying to process all that has happened and come to terms with the new reality. It is the natural process of recovery. Talk these feelings out with loved ones, fellow sufferers or with a good therapist.

## Filling in the Gaps and Moving On
The second year of recovery.

By the time a year has passed most people are pulling their lives together although few would say they are the same people they were before their illness.

Physically, most have come to terms with the healing process, have learnt how to pace themselves and are enjoying a slow but steady progress. They have had several medical check ups and they are beginning to feel more confident about the future. However, experiencing a life threatening event, be it illness or trauma, can have deep reaching consequences.

When you were ill; in order to survive you had to strip away all the unnecessary "stuff". On the simplest level, time has now passed and the little things you worried about then have either resolved themselves or you simply don't care any more.

Staring death in the face changes things and an awareness of wanting more can grow. One realises that life is short, fragile, and can end abruptly. You may feel that simply getting along day after day is not enough anymore.

Everyone needs to find their own answers. Some people look to conventional religion, others need to look further.

Read books, talk to like minded people, follow your heart. Who knows where it will lead and what life purpose you will find?
It is reported that The Dalai Lama, when asked what surprised him most about humanity, answered;

*"Man. Because he sacrifices his health to make money. Then he sacrifices money to recuperate his health. And then he is so anxious about the future that he does not enjoy the present; the result being that he does not live in the present or the future; he lives as if he is never going to die, and then dies having never really lived."*

Perhaps this has been a "wake-up" call and the best is yet to come.

# 5.
# Caring for loved ones

## Caring for your Spouse/Partner

Finding out that your Partner has cancer is a terrible thing. It can be likened to suddenly finding yourself an "Also Ran" in a race you never wanted to enter in the first place. You are not the "lead runner" but you are also running very very hard. Please read the receiving bad news chapter because you are just as deeply affected by all of this.

As the wife/husband/partner you are in a very difficult supportive role. Whereas the patient will get all the attention – you will get very little or none. Most will expect you to just carry on, keep the job going, run your household and family, visit the hospital and be optimistic at all times. Through ignorance we have become a harsh and intolerant society.

The real story is that you both now are experiencing this illness and you are equally as upset as your loved one. Your life has changed too. Your hopes and dreams are equally effected with the added prospect of, perhaps, someday, being left behind.

It is normal to feel the "anger that must never be spoken of," a type of survivors guilt and resentment.

Your partner may have to actively experience this illness and the treatments, but you are here too, trying your best to be upbeat and cope. This can be a very lonely place. Everyone who has supported a loved one through illness has experienced these challenges and feelings. You are just being human and these feelings will need to be addressed.

The most healthy way through is always communication and planning. Trying to ignore what is going on is simply "tip toeing around the elephant in the room". Everybody knows it's there. Try to discuss these things from day one, it will only get harder the longer you leave it as each tries not to upset the other. This is still your lover and partner. He/she is feeling all these things as well. Discussing realities has never shortened a life yet but it has lengthened many. Plan for the "what if's". Even the bad ones – they may never come to pass.

When you find yourself in this position others, perhaps those you never expected, will come out of the background to support you. Many will have been there themselves and have valuable coping strategies to share and you in your turn will help others.

Accepting help and admitting to our vulnerabilities is difficult for many people. This is a long road and can be very lonely if you do not allow benevolent others into your life.

There will be difficult times ahead but if approached correctly they can bring you closer to an ever deepening state of love and understanding making you both stronger and better able to face the future.

Just as your partner needs to plan for the times ahead, so must you.

It is very unlikely you ever liked to be together 24/7, so it is even more unlikely either of you will be able to tolerate it now! Just as your loved one needs a sanctuary to rest and recover you too will need time out. It is important to get out and interact with your friends and be "normal" if even just for a little time. This will make you both feel better and give you something to talk about later. So, before things get difficult, plan your escapes.

Perhaps coffee every Saturday morning or golf with the lads as usual. Take the time to have your evenings out for hobbies and interests, go to the gym and look after the garden / children / grandchildren / pets as normal. Remember, your loved one will require a lot of quiet time to heal, you do not need to be there all the time. Create your sanctuary in the home where you too can be comfortable and relaxed and not "on top of each other".

Just as with your partner, hard times are no excuse for neglecting yourself and letting personal standards go. It takes effort to keep your identity during this time when you are physically and emotionally exhausted but it will pay off.

## Mental health

What is good for the goose is good for the gander. The strategies discussed in the mental health section will help you as well. You are in this together and all the new insights your partner experiences you will too. Life has now irrevocably changed, but as you progress through this and allow changes to occur, you will find strengths you never knew you had, meet amazing people who will come into your life to help and come to a deeper understanding of life and love.

## Coping with others

There are two types of people, those who help and those who don't. Those who don't can be very troubling and critical.

If you are lucky your boss will be sympathetic, but this is not always the case and can be very stressful. There is not really a lot one can do in this case except the obvious and jobs can be hard to find! Try to plan your leave around the most crucial periods such as return from hospital for a few days and post chemotherapy.

Cancer volunteers are very helpful taking people to and from appointments and it will also help keep your loved one from becoming too dependant, as when we are with strangers one has to make an effort – and this is no bad thing when fighting to keep ones identity through an illness.

Other members of the family and friends might be able to help as well which will make them feel involved. Your job is important and a necessary income during this troubled time.

Of course everyone has an opinion, and it's often critical of you. It is, sadly, human nature to lash out when one feels upset and powerless. One cannot upset the ill person, so who is next? Although it is an understandable reaction it is still not acceptable.

A good coping strategy is to compile and rehearse your ideal answer so that when the critical comment comes, usually when you least expect it, you can just trot an answer out, then go home and remove them from the Christmas card list!

Some suggestions are;

*"Say that again?"* People rarely have to courage to repeat a nasty comment when you look at then full in the face.

*"Are you trying to make me feel bad?"*

*"During this difficult time I really don't have energy to waste on negativity."*

Relatives can be another difficult area and avoidance strategies are called for. A good tip is to change their ring tone so that you are never caught unaware.

In-Laws need to be helpful or absent. Yes, they are suffering too and it must be dreadful see your child ill, but they cannot take it out on you, the primary carer.

Discuss this with your loved one and ask how often and how they want to see their parents. Few of us want to be babied or fussed over. Then be firm, not cruel, just firm.

There is an etiquette for visiting, hospital and home that is discussed later in this book. Diversionary tactics for the more persistent include playing the immunity protection card – "The Doctor says no visitors until the immune system picks up" – and the old blood pressure one, two – raised blood pressure, the Doctor says total rest. These are often true and at the very least you are acting in a preventative role!

However, if your loved one really wants to see the awful relatives and you find them caustic, you might just need to leave a tray with cake and go out thanking them profusely for giving you the opportunity to do much needed "chores" as you rush past them in the doorway, and then go and do something nice.

Modern day families are complicated with children and exes. Emotions can run high. Everyone knows their own circumstances and family best. Take advice, talk to sympathetic members and enlist their help. As the partner, you will find yourself "on the front line". There is no easy way through this but try to be kind and remember , you did not make this happen.

Talking to children is heartbreaking for all. Try to be as honest and simple as possible. They will ask a lot of questions and you will find books, literature and advisers available to help from cancer charities and on the internet. You do not always need to be strong. Crying together allows children to express their upset as well as showing them you are upset too. Family counselling can also be very helpful at this time.

**Caring for your parent.**

Finding out that a parent has cancer is a terrible blow. No matter what your relationship is, good or bad, it is a shock and often our first real hit of mortality. It makes us feel vulnerable because the "buffer" we had between us and the great unknown might be compromised.

Many emotions flood in and, even if not on good terms, the person who gave you half your genes, who is, at a basic level, half you, may be leaving. If you are lucky to be close, you may well be losing one of the few people in life who love and support you simply because you are you. It is one step closer to standing as an adult, alone and responsible, no matter what your age.

So, you too, will be very upset and angry. It is a life change thrust upon you without your consent. It will never come at a good time, we are all so busy. Time will be needed to support your family and explanations may need to be made to children on uncomfortable topics, see above.

All of these and more are natural feelings. We are not machines, but human beings with emotions, and some of our strongest emotions revolve around our parents who made us and reared us.

As always communication is the key. Try to talk to your partner or friends so that these feelings can be expressed and dealt with.

However, please remember that no matter how difficult it might be, it is natural for children to outlive their parents. Something all of us have to face at some stage in our lives. To lose one's partner, however, is much more painful thing. So, when you interact with your parent(s), their partner and/or step parents please be mindful that this is their show and they get to choose how to deal with it.

You may not agree, but it is not your call. Try to be respectful of their decisions and learn from their actions. If nothing else you may decide that this route is one you would never take and it will help you to plan for future "What If's". As roughly one person in three in our society is affected by cancer, you may well get your chance to handle things better later.

Not all families have an open and frank relationship, in fact very few do. It is very likely that issues from childhood will bubble to the surface. They say there is no such thing as a happy childhood and all of us have some issues from along the way. Try not to bury these. It is better to "bring them to the table" where you can ponder them and decide what action, if any, is necessary. Talk to trusted loved ones and, if troubled by anger, find a good therapist. A family row at this time will help no one.

# 6.
# VISITING ETIQUETTE

The bottom line here is ask the principal carer if they would like you to visit. Often people are very ill, or weak, or in quarantine due to immunity issues and visiting is not appropriate just then. Other people just do not want to be seen in a vulnerable state. If this is so, a card with a handwritten note, or the offer of help will be most appreciated.

Remember, the partner needs support too, and the invite to a coffee or some practical help can be a life line. Even the odd chat on the 'phone. If a visit is welcome, you may be able to take the place of the principal carer and give them a break.

## When visiting someone in hospital

Nowadays there is little hospital visiting as people are discharged home as soon as possible. If you wish to visit remember this person is ill enough to be in hospital and therefore weak and vulnerable. Some basic guidelines are;

- Prepare yourself not to show shock, they will not be looking their best.

- No more than two by the bedside. If someone else comes, leave as soon as possible.

- Keep your visit short, no more than twenty minutes, ten is better. Even if it's going well, they are making a big effort to be sociable and using valuable energy needed for healing. Remember the old adage, always leave them wanting more!

- Do not cross talk over the bed. This is exhausting for the patient. If you want to chat with another visitor meet after, perhaps for a coffee in the hospital cafe.

- Space is tight. So if you bring anything, make it small such as a card that they can look at later. Many hospitals have banned flowers and food treats just spoil, so keep those for later when they can appreciate them at home.

- Talk slowly as an ill person's brain is very busy getting better and might also be fuzzy with drugs.

- Keep to upbeat topics. You are trying to empower them, not depress them!

**When visiting a close relative**

There is nothing more comforting than having your loved ones visit and share time with you, and that is the purpose of visiting. You are not expected to entertain, just be.

Of course it is your job to bring fresh laundry and treats as required. Nice music selections and messages from family members which can be replayed are especially welcome.

**Helpful stuff to do**

Help with self care. Even the best hospitals rarely have time for more than the most basic grooming. Help with hair, make up, shaving, oral hygiene and nails can really boost morale.

Massage

A hand or foot massage is so loving and relaxing. IV lines are often in situ. and hands can get uncomfortably stiff also, increased contact with the bedsheets makes skin uncomfortably dry. There is no need for specialist oils, hand cream is fine. Use enough to comfortably glide over the skin with a firm but gentle pressure and simply avoid involved areas such as drip sites.

Reading aloud.

In the days before modern medicine and people took a long time to recover, it was traditional to read aloud when sitting with a loved one. This is a skill we now rarely use, but it is worth giving it a go as it allows them to truly relax without having to think. Listening to a loved ones voice makes us feel cherished and loved. Many drift off into the best of healing sleeps.

Newspaper, poetry or books, whichever you both enjoy. Just sitting at a bedside can be awkward and stressful for you both, but reading helps time pass in a pleasant way.

## Visiting in ICU

Your loved on may be in intensive care post operation or following stem cell treatment. Stem cell treatment requires a very controlled environment because the existing stem cells will have been destroyed to kill the cancer and new ones need to be introduced. This means the immune system has been temporarily destroyed and it needs to re-establish. It is therefore very important to prevent infection, so isolation and barrier nursing is required. This means just the closest relatives and strict visiting rules where everybody must gown up and wear masks.

ICU is a scary place for everyone. There will be IV's and various monitoring machines bleeping and whirring. Everything is harsh and pristine with display lights and occasional alarms going off. Fortunately, the patient will sleep through most of this as their body is in deep healing mode.

We are not allowed to bring much into this environment, but there is a little you can do to make it more comfortable. It is a proven fact that nature makes us feel better, even looking at it. A beautiful paper picture put where it can be easily viewed, but not in the way, gives a lovely focal point for your loved one to concentrate on and provide a measure of escape from the present.

A nice piece of rose quartz can be suitably cleansed and very comforting, see Healing Crystals.

Music is always our friend and earphones placed under the pillow slip easy to listen to. An eye mask will be appreciated and a relaxing aromatherapy spray to spritz the pillow slip can also aid relaxation.

## Visiting at Home

Recovering from cancer treatment as already discussed is a long process. As a relative or close friend you will be keen to see your loved one, especially if prevented whilst they were in hospital. However, please remember to respect the principal carer's wishes; they know the situation and are only trying to protect your loved from exhaustion and harm. There will be time later when your input will be most appreciated as they improve and strength returns.

Preparation
Before your visit prepare yourself to be a calm state of mind. The appearance of your loved one may have changed, so prepare yourself for a shock and try not to show it. Have a couple of nice uncomplicated topics to talk about and speak in quiet measured way. Remember, the patient's brain is very busy healing and probably a bit fuzzy with medication. The time for humour and jokes will come later.

How long is long enough?  This will increase as recovery progresses. Ask the principal carer. Getting better is boring and tedious. It can be so lovely to see a friend with news of the outside world that one forgets just how much energy this takes and tired one will be later.

Have an exit strategy planned, and just be honest. "I'm popping in just for a short time to see how you are and let you know I/we are thinking of you". Remember, no matter how good they look, they are putting on a show for you and will be secretly relieved when they can rest again. It is the fact that you have physically visited that matters, not the duration. Gentle hand holding and a kiss to the cheek if appropriate.

On leaving, an offer of another visit, a phone call, or when appropriate, a simple outing to look forward to as their strength returns, will give everyone something nice to look forward to.

Gifts to bring - Flowers, an interesting book or film and treats will be welcomed. A good practical gift is a selection of ready meals either home made or bought. A short video is easily compiled and messages from the children, friendship circle, or simply a film of a favourite walk or a place of beauty are very uplifting and can be viewed again during the dark times.

# ABOUT THE AUTHOR

Gillian Howell is a life long healer. Growing up in Northern Ireland during the "troubles"and frustrated by helplessness Gillian walked out of school mid term at seventeen years of age to become a nurse in a major Belfast Hospital, then a midwife and finally a Health Visitor where she practiced in inner city Belfast during the height of the conflict.

Due to her husband's occupation, Gillian and their three children travelled extensively. Fascinated with all aspects of healing Gillian further studied aromatherapy, hypnotherapy, NLP and then qualified as a Homeopathic Doctor. She now lives with her husband in Cornwall.